AF198656

Green Coffee - A weight loss guarantee?

How you can lose weight quickly and easily with green coffee

Peter Carl Simons

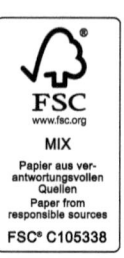

Bibliografische Information der Deutschen Nationalbibliothek:

Die Deutsche Nationalbibliothek verzeichnet diese Publikation in der Deutschen Nationalbibliografie; detaillierte bibliografische Daten sind im Internet über http://dnb.dnb.de abrufbar.

Herstellung und Verlag: BoD – Books on Demand, Norderstedt

ISBN: 978-3-7519-2116-9

Introduction

By using this book, you accept this disclaimer in full.

No advice

The book contains information. The information is not advice and should not be treated as such.

No representations or warranties

To the maximum extent permitted by applicable law and subject to section below, we exclude all representations, warranties, undertakings and guarantees relating to the book.

Without prejudice to the generality of the foregoing paragraph, we do not represent, warrant, undertake or guarantee:

- that the information in the book is correct, accurate, complete or non-misleading.

- that the use of the guidance in the book will lead to any particular outcome or result.

Limitations and exclusions of liability

The limitations and exclusions of liability set out in this section and elsewhere in this disclaimer: are subject to section 6 below; and govern all liabilities arising under the disclaimer or in relation to the book, including liabilities arising in contract, in tort (including negligence) and for breach of statutory duty.

We will not be liable to you in respect of any losses arising out of any event or events beyond our reasonable control.

We will not be liable to you in respect of any business losses, including without limitation loss of or damage to profits, income, revenue, use, production, anticipated savings, business, contracts, commercial opportunities or goodwill.

We will not be liable to you in respect of any loss or corruption of any data, database or software.

We will not be liable to you in respect of any special, indirect or consequential loss or damage.

Exceptions

Nothing in this disclaimer shall: limit or exclude our liability for death or personal injury resulting from negligence; limit or exclude our liability for fraud or fraudulent misrepresentation; limit any of our liabilities in any way that is not permitted under applicable law; or exclude any of our liabilities that may not be excluded under applicable law.

Severability

If a section of this disclaimer is determined by any court or other competent authority to be unlawful and/or unenforceable, the other sections of this disclaimer continue in effect.

If any unlawful and/or unenforceable section would be lawful or enforceable if part of it were deleted, that part will be deemed to be deleted, and the rest of the section will continue in effect.

Law and jurisdiction

This disclaimer will be governed by and construed in accordance with Swiss law, and any disputes relating to this disclaimer will be subject to the exclusive jurisdiction of the courts of Switzerland.

Inhaltsverzeichnis

Inhaltsverzeichnis **9**

Preface **11**

We need a modern diet **13**

Green Coffee **15**

Effects *17*

Preparation *19*

Using it every day - What can you expect? *21*

Warning and contraindication *23*

Success factors for your target weight **26**

Finally **27**

Preface

As soon as one diet trend has lost its momentum, the industry throws another one at you. That can be seen especially on teleshopping channels and online markets. After artichoke and pineapple products were offered virtually everywhere, green coffee extract seems to start taking their place. Already you can buy it in capsules, powders, pills, and even in double filter bags.

What all these offers have in common is the unnecessary production step between the green, unroasted coffee beans, and the offered product. A product that would cost about 2-3 Euros per kilo (world market price) thus quickly becomes 60 capsules with 400mg extract each, at, believe it or not, 15 Euros. That makes for 600 Euros of profit for 1 kg of coffee extract.

While it is correct that one kilo of coffee doesn't equal one kilo of coffee extract, and the product has to be packaged as well, common sense inadvertently concludes that whoever offers the extract must make considerable profits with it.

There are actually several scientific studies that provide evidence for the positive influence of green coffee for body weight and health. If you take a closer look at these studies, however, you will find that these positive effects can not be attributed to the compressed extract, but that they can be achieved by consuming green coffee just as well, if you are doing it right. This knowledge, that my former employers were keen on keeping undisclosed, is what I am offering to you, dear readers, in this publication.

If you, too, want to work against the money-making with miracle cures, and rather prefer honest information, I would appreciate some feedback online, and recommendations to other people with weight problems.

Thank you for that

Sincerely, Peter Carl Simons

We need a modern diet

In our quite mobile society, unhealthy foods are almost a necessary evil for many people. Many need to get their lunch in cafeterias that put more value on "cheap" than on "healthy". Others often don't even get the chance to eat regularly or healthily due to field work, shift work or similar arrangements. More and more foods with unhealthy additives and sugars do their part in fattening the society.

It is not surprising that many manufacturers that produce these unhealthy and fattening foods also start offering dietary products or calory-reduced foods. This way they can make more money by correcting the results of malnutrition partly stemming from ingredients of their own products. A classic case of profiting twice. It probably won't be long until a well-known drink with lots of sugar in it will come with a coupon for a sample of the dietary product made by the same manufacturer.

Loosing weight is a billion-dollar business, and the revenue and profit forecasts for this sector are on a perpetual rise.[1]

And actually, there is an alternative that is largely body-friendly, entirely natural - even available in organic quality - and extremely inexpensive. You can calculate about 10-20 Euros per month that you will get back through omitting the corresponding amount of roasted coffee.

---

[1] If you want to invest some more money - this market provides above-average profits, and a perpetually growing market.)

Green Coffee

Contrary to what you may thing, "green coffee" doesn't mean organic coffee, but simply coffee that has not been roasted. Hence it isn't brown, but slightly green or beige. That means we are talking about the natural beans before they are roasted into coffee by roasting plants - or by some enthusiasts at home - that is then offered in grocery stores.

Green coffee, other than roasted coffee beans, still contains all the healthy ingredients that are partly destroyed by the roasting process.

In terms of taste, green coffee is somewhat similar to usual coffee. Personally, the taste of green coffee kind of reminds me a bit of herbal tea.

The green coffee extract that I had mentioned before, by the way, is nothing but brewed green coffee that has been steam-dried.

Which means that in the best case it contains the very same active ingredients that you can get by brewing green coffee yourself for a fraction of the price - on top of that fresh and tasty. If the steam-dry process wasn't done carefully enough though, this means less active ingredients for you, and essentially paying more, for less effect.

Effects

While burning fat, chlorogenic acid is quite important[2]. It provides the basis of the fat-burning effect of green coffee. After roasting, however, this active ingredient is largely destroyed.

---

2 Wikipedia.de states about this active ingredient: "(...) Chlorogenic acid showed effects on biological systems in various studies. It is notable that this is an effect proven by scientific studies, that are, however, not to be understood as medical effects. To make this kind of statement, further and more thorough research would have to be conducted.

Chlorogenic acid is a well-known antioxidant that protects the DNA from damage with its isomers - an effect that was evident even against damages due to nuclear radiation. It slows the absorbtion of sugar into the blood after a meal. This is evidence for an antidiabetic effect of chlorogenic acid in animal tests. Additionally, the effect of blood pressure reduction was noted in humans. Chlorogenic acid reduces platelet aggregation (blood clotting). Animal testing with Swiss mice (laboratory mice) showed positive effects against various stomach ulcer models. It could be shown that chlorogenic acid can reduce liver inflammation. A cellular model showed that chlorogenic acid is able to invoke apoptosis (programmed cell death) for cancer cells.")

In simple terms, one could write that chlorogenic acid significantly limits the body's ability to absorb and store sugar. If the body can not store enough sugar anymore, this automatically reduces the storing of fat. The body is required to use its fat reserves in order to keep functioning. The result of a continuous ingestion of green coffee thus means the continuous loss of body fat percentage, and thereby a loss of weight.

This effect even works without being substituted by sports or changing your diet. Needless to say, however, that changing the diet as well as increasing activity are also important in the context of healthy weight loss.

Preparation

The first challenge when preparing green coffee is grinding it. Other than the relatively brittle roasted coffee beans, green coffee is quite hard and contains a lot of residual moisture, which is why it is hard to grind.

One single try with a manual coffee grinder or the mill of a common coffee machine may lead to a complete failure. I had the best success with heavy-duty mills with rotating fly cutters, as they are used for grinding nuts as well. Fortunately more and more green coffee manufacturers also provide grinded green coffee. Such grinded greed coffee is currently offered on the internet for less than 20 Euros per kilo. As smaller volumes are also available, there is not really a good reason against trying yourself.

The actual preparation of green coffee is, after all, not that hard.

Just grind the raw coffee fine or coarse, depending on your preference - you can just test what tastes best for you - or simply buy pre-grinded green coffee beans.

Depending on your taste, put the desired amount of grinded coffee into a coffee filter (as you probably know it from "normal" filter coffee), and pour hot water over it.

Alternatively you can simply put the grinded raw coffee into a cup and pour hot water over it. Leave it for 10 minutes, and then filter out the stock with a fine sieve.

It is recommended not to sweeten green coffee too much if you are aiming at losing weight. If you are not looking for weight loss, it can be sweetened just like any other coffee.

Of course it is much easier to just carry some capsules or pills with you instead of brewing your fresh green coffee everywhere.

Fortunately, that is not necessary at all. You can simply brew your coffee in the morning, or in the evening before, and just take it with you and drink it over the course of the day.

Regardless of whether you want to reduce your weight with green coffee extract or self-brewed green coffee: Don't expect any miracles. Reliable studies were largely conducted over a course of 4-6 months, and most participants not only showed a significant loss in weight, but also an overall increase in health.

I personally know people who had drank 3-5 cups of green coffee a day instead of normal coffee, and managed to lose ten kilos in two months. Nowadays they largely avoid "normal" coffee in favour of their new favourite drink.

None of them have changed anything else about their life.

Warning and contraindication

In general one could say that every person who can drink "normal" coffee, may enjoy green coffee in the same amounts. As green coffee contains less caffeine than roasted coffee, this is hardly a problem.

In any case, people suffering from illnesses or morbid obesity should consult their doctor about any change in diet.

Green coffee is not suited for the following people:

- Pregnant and breastfeeding women,

- People with caffeine-intolerance,

- People suffering from diabetes, high blood pressure, and circulatory problems,

- Children,

- People who can not tolerate roasted coffee for some reason.

There is no good recommendation to give on the minimal and maximum amount of green coffee one should drink each day. Depending on your body weight and your overall health as well as the strength of the coffee, various factors play a role. Generally, consuming green coffee as a substitute for the same amount of roasted coffee is no problem at all.

A health-threatening overdose is hardly achievable with green coffee, if you drink it. An overdose of chlorogenic acid could be achieved after consuming (depending on the source) 5-10 litres of green coffee a day. Such quantities, however, make no sense at all though. People who were successful with weight loss by consuming green coffee approximately consumed one litre a day.

If after the consumption of green coffee you should note one or more of the following side effects, you should cease consumption and contact a doctor:

- Tachycardia,

- Unrest,

- Sleeplessness,

- Discomfort.

Success factors for your target weight

In the context of weight reduction you surely have to distinguish between people who do it for aesthetic reasons, or just to attain their "bikini body" or their "sixpack". For them, the consumption of a few cups of green coffee per day is generally the best method to achieve their dream weight and to keep it.

People with morbid obesity, however, should consult their doctor. it is especially important to consider that most cases of morbid obesity include some psychological reasons. Check whether it is possible to get help from a coach or a psychologist.

Any weight loss is easier and quicker, if it is combined with a change in diet, and an increase in activity. That doesn't need to be extreme sports. Even a daily evening stroll or similar measures can be a step in the right direction.

Finally

Other than many guidebook authors, I am neither offering the products of certain manufacturers, nor is it my intention to advertise for anyone. Other than the modest fee for this book, I am not making any profit from sharing my experience with you. As it is very important to me to share this knowledge and this weight loss approach, I would be thankful if you could give me some feedback online - as well as your own experiences with green coffee.

All information contained in this book are in accordance with my own experiences and my own research. They are not to be seen as instructions, or as a substitute for expert consultation.